FREE TO BE

FREE TO BE

THE NON-DIET PATH TO PEACE
WITH FOOD AND BODY

ASHLEY HEINTZELMAN, PHD
SHANA ARNHOLD MPA, PA-C

Table of Contents

Forward   1

Introduction   3

Free to Be Tools   13

    Tool 1: Change Your Goals   15

    Tool 2: Focus on Values, Not your Appearance   18

    Tool 3: Learn about Your Relationship with Food 21

    Tool 4: When you Want to Eat, but you're NOT Hungry 23

    Tool 5: Studying Yourself after you Eat   26

    Tool 6: Prioritize Self-Care   29

    Tool 7: Practice Self-Compassion   36

    Tool 8: Expectations for the Process   38

Closing Thoughts   41

Food Peace Worksheet   43

FAQs and Resources   48

Citations   57

Forward

Negative body image plagues millions of men, women, and even children every day. The number on the scale has the power to dictate their mood, self-esteem and behaviors. With fear of the so-called "obesity epidemic" hanging over their heads, people grasp at all sorts of methods to try and control their weight, often in the name of "health." Yet people often use all sorts of unhealthy (and unsustainable) behaviors to produce weight loss.

The data is clear: dieting doesn't work. It might produce temporary weight loss, but the studies consistently show that the weight lost will be regained (often plus some) within 2-5 years. The cycle of yo-yo dieting tends to ratchet weight up over time, leaving the person more and more desperate for the faulty promises of the weight loss industry. This constant fluctuation in weight is, in itself, harmful to the body, promoting the very health conditions that dieting sought to prevent. The dieting industry is sold on pseudoscience and lies, and it preys on people's insecurities.

In addition to the detrimental impact on physical health, dieting does psychological harm as well. It teaches people to disconnect from their bodies. After all, if you could trust your hunger and fullness cues, why would you need to diet in the first place? Tricks of the trade include things like counting calories, grams or points. It's also common to have lists of foods that are acceptable and unacceptable. Then there's the magic potions of shakes, powders, pills and supplements that claim to rev up metabolism, burn fat, or squash hunger. At best these products are a complete waste of money; and at worst they are outright dangerous, and some have been known to cause damage to the body. To me, however, the most detrimental aspect of dieting is the way it erodes a person's self-esteem and trust with their body.

The good news in all of this? There is a revolution taking place. Healthcare providers are realizing that dieting doesn't work and that the health-related claims related to weight have been far over exaggerated. There is a movement taking place that is anti-dieting and about listening to your body instead. Size and weight diversity are starting to be recognized and accepted, along with a push towards body positivity and self-compassion. Now don't get me wrong, the dieting industry still makes billions of dollars per year and size bias and weight discrimination are still pervasive issues, but strides are being made to change the status quo.

In this book, *Free to Be: The non-diet path to peace with food and body*, Ashley and Shana take a scientifically sound and fiercely compassionate perspective on ditching dieting for good. Coming from backgrounds in medicine and psychology, they are a dynamic duo in terms of helping the reader understand what it means to have a healthy relationship with food and your body.

They outline the many ways diet culture shows up in our lives, and the ways diets work against us. They walk you through how to change the way you think about food, weight and exercise. Each section includes practical action steps that will give you clarity as you walk through this process. Their approach brings together the current evidence-based and best practices in the fields of psychology and medicine. THIS is the path toward healing your relationship with food and your body. I hope you enjoy this book as much as I did. It's sure to be a resource that you can revisit time and time again, and one that you'll want to share with many others in your life.

Katy Harvey, MS, RD, LD, CEDRD, is a non-diet dietitian who specializes in the treatment of eating disorders, negative body image, emotional eating and chronic dieting

Introduction

YOU CAN ABSOLUTELY ENJOY FOOD, STOP
OBSESSING AND FEEL WELL!

Phew, we had to get that out there right away. But there's a catch, there's always a catch. You have to ditch the food rules. All of them. Because rules = diets, and by now you know the truth: diets don't work. In the short-term you may feel well and lose some weight, but you're also spending waaaay too much time calculating, weighing, and thinking (fantasizing?) about food, as well as avoiding friends, ignoring body signals and certainly not living the life you want. Long-term, well, you know how it ends. Ahem, regain the weight (plus some usually), with all the self-loathing that comes along with the pounds. And why would anyone want to "get healthy" only short-term?

For the purposes of our book, we're defining a "diet" as a rule-based form of eating with the goal of weight loss. The diet rules may be related to what, when, or how much you're "allowed" to eat.

If you are a chronic dieter or preoccupied with food or weight, you are not alone.

- o 45% of adults say they are preoccupied with their weight some or all of the time.[1]
- o 65% of the 4,023 American women between the ages of 25 and 45 surveyed reported having disordered eating behaviors, and 74.5% reported that concerns about their weight and shape interfered with their happiness.[2]

Even more eye-opening is that fact that if you spend more than 30% of your total conscious time thinking about food or your body (what to eat or not eat, worrying or guilt about food, etc.), many eating disorder specialists consider this meeting criteria for an eating disorder. It is considered a disorder given the degree of psychological distress that comes from spending so many of your waking hours thinking about food or your body. That really illustrates the seriousness of the issue, doesn't it?

No matter where you are on the spectrum of food-related issues, your life as it relates to food is likely governed by rules, so many ever-changing rules. Why? Because you want a plan that will finally change things. Having these strict guidelines addresses some needs for you, like autonomy, purpose, companionship, maybe even distraction from other emotional issues. It feels good to have the promise of weight loss and happiness, and you feel empowered (for a moment). But when that fleeting moment is gone, it may not be long until you latch onto or at least strongly consider the next diet craze. Because you just haven't found the RIGHT program for you, right? No, my friend, but the bazillon-dollar diet industry has tricked us into believing this and now you're TIRED.

Tired of spending so much time and energy focused on what to eat or not to eat

Tired of isolating yourself when on a diet

Tired of worrying about your weight and how your clothes will fit

Tired of trying to control your mind and body or feeling out of control around food

Tired of spending money on the next best thing

Tired of judging and maybe even hating yourself over food choices

Tired of mistrusting yourself

Tired of emotional eating

Tired of the "lose/gain" or "all in/all out" cycle

Tired of feeling like a failure after another diet attempt

Tired of disrespecting your body

Tired of guilt surrounding food

Tired of putting off something you really want to do until you lose weight

Tired of your negative relationship with food affecting other parts of your life

Tired of feeling hopeless that you can make lasting changes

Tired of counting calories, and self-imposed food restrictions

Tired of punishing yourself mentally or physically for eating something "bad"

Does this sound familiar? You are physically, mentally and emotionally exhausted—and we haven't even touched on the other stressful aspects of life like relationships, kids, work and family. Stress is the real enemy here (or should be, as it's much more a factor in poor health than health behaviors), and we are ADDING to our stress by creating food rules for ourselves! The stress of a diet in many ways is getting you further from what you want regarding improved health, body acceptance or weight normalization.

Restricting food has both psychological and physiological effects. It gives the "off-limits" food power and charm, often leading to cravings, overeating or bingeing. Even rats overeat when deprived of food. The best way to ensure obsessive thoughts about food? Start a diet.

> The best way to ensure obsessive thoughts about food?
> Start a diet.

What if you could use all that time, energy and money on something else? Invest it in yourself and your family? Take a moment to imagine a life in which you truly are NOT WORRIED about food or your body. You enjoy eating and are at peace with yourself. Think about how liberating that could be! We want to help you get there.

We are medical professionals with the knowledge and experience to help get you to that place. Ashley Heintzelman, PhD, is a Licensed Psychologist and Eating Disorder Specialist with years of experience treating patients with the same problems you have. She knows what works because **this is what she does every day.**

Shana Arnhold is a Physician Assistant in Gastroenterology with a background in kinesiology. As a former restrictive eater preoccupied with food and weight, she has been able to overcome the struggle with food and free herself from this detrimental cycle. She counsels patients regarding weight struggles on a regular basis and has come to believe the medical model is all wrong—focusing on weight and trying to control our actions (what we're eating, how much we're moving, etc.) instead of **listening to our bodies and addressing underlying issues.**

Inspiration Behind This Book and Why It's Unique

In our daily work, we see people who are miserable in their bodies, preoccupied with food, and/or always trying to lose weight. We also see the divide between professional psychological therapy, which many don't end up seeking, and conventional medicine, which lacks the tools to adequately address what's really causing the struggle for so many. **This book aims to bridge that gap.**

To help people make peace with food and body, we've created a summary of recommendations based on our own professional experiences as well as the elements of the existing non-diet literature that we have found to be most beneficial. This book is a collection of tools and information that we have found to be the most valuable and helpful for positive change, packaged in a clear and concise way that you can use to get to work applying to your daily life. We certainly encourage you to dive deeper into the topics that are most relevant to your journey.

How Did I Get Here?

Why is this happening? Why do we keep searching for the next quick fix? It's complex and multifaceted for everyone. Your relationship with food and your body comes from the intersection of many factors, including cultural messages, the way your family discussed and treated food and body image, your genetic makeup and your unique personal life experiences.

Diet Culture

Diet culture is a societal system of beliefs about food and weight that promotes thinness and restrictive eating. It encompasses the diet industry, weight loss supplement and pharmaceutical industries, beauty industry, media and marketing, as well as your personal experiences. These can all work together to make us feel inadequate and undesirable, motivating us to spend more time and money on the next fad.

The diet industry alone makes billions of dollars per year by making you believe that you will be happier if you tone, tweak or shrink your body. It literally banks off of our insecurities, and it's toxic!

Diet culture tends to disparage those who do don't align with what's considered "healthy," almost deeming the favored behaviors honorable or moral.[3] It is so pervasive and insidious that it seems completely normal to be putting your effort into changing yourself versus accepting or enjoying yourself as you are. It's ingrained in us before our adolescence, being passed down from people who have never been taught to reject it. Think of events such as planning a wedding, going on a beach vacation or even having a baby. So many of those happy experiences are overshadowed by focusing on losing weight before or after the event. We are taught to conform to the diet culture that leads us to believe that our experiential satisfaction is tied to our weight and we are being robbed of our joy in the meantime.

We are taught to conform to the diet culture that leads us to believe that our experiential satisfaction is tied to our weight and we are being robbed of our joy in the meantime.

Examples of diet culture:

- Magazine articles about changing one's body
- Rigid eating patterns
- Counting calories
- Equating thinness with health
- "Cleanses"
- Labeling food as good or bad
- Exercise as punishment
- Comments made about someone's body or weight (intended as positive or negative)
- Discrimination based on weight
- Lack of representation for a variety of body types
- Millions of posts on Instagram promoting "fit" bodies

It is difficult not to get sucked in, it's everywhere! In the end, you can't change what other people do, but you CAN learn to individually recognize and reject diet culture.

How Did I Get Here? Mental aspects

Emotional eating and habits

Simply put, emotional eating is using food to help yourself feel better. Sometimes we eat due to an uncomfortable feeling such as boredom, worry or feeling unappreciated. However, emotional eating doesn't necessarily mean feeling upset or stressed and burying your feelings in your favorite comfort food. It can be much more insidious or hard to recognize, such as an underlying but not openly apparent reason for overeating or "filling a void." How about a fun social situation? If you are restricting food regularly, this is a time when it's easy to "let go" and overeat.

Sometimes food is a nonjudgmental, dependable tactic to distract from or cope with what we're really feeling. Eating temporarily calms our motions; wanting to eat when we're not hungry is a sign of a need, and not necessarily a bad thing, but it becomes problematic when it's our primary coping mechanism. Eating when our system doesn't need it may be followed by guilt and sometimes weight gain (further evidence of your "failure" and further propagating the negative cycle).

Many people say they come home from work and eat in front of the television just because it's a routine, not necessarily in response to a negative feeling. Eating may be an unconscious habit or a way to "zone out" and relax after a long day.

We can learn to recognize our own patterns and be curious about and accepting of what we are feeling. Being in touch with feelings, self-respect, and kindness—NOT self-control will lead to less emotional or unconscious eating.

We're drawn to diets because they provide structure, streamline decision-making and can provide quick (though temporary) results. But remember that adhering to a certain regime only perpetuates the diet mentality, and we know that <u>diets don't lead to long-term body satisfaction or sustained weight normalization.</u> Both our bodies and psyche reject the limits put on food variety, calories, etc. We will discuss this and the need for a consistent mentality shift in more detail to come.

Inescapability

Food is such a big part of our lives and can't be avoided like smoking or other addictions. That's why it's so important to <u>do the work</u> and change the way we view food—as a neutral object which is not inherently good or bad. Across cultures, food often represents nurturing, connection, celebration, comfort, reward and family time. No wonder our relationship with food is so complicated and we are drawn to a diet that promises simple rules for weight loss! Our goal is to help you have a more relaxed feeling and approach toward food, helping to decrease your stress responses surrounding food and gatherings. This book is about much more than food—our goal is to help you get back to enjoying time with your family and friends and **savoring your life**.

How Did I Get Here? Physical Aspects

Your body has physiologic mechanisms in place to maintain homeostasis (weight stability). One example is that dieting triggers a reduction in leptin, the hormone responsible for satiety. This results in increased appetite. Chronic dieting leads to chronically suppressed leptin and metabolic tendencies to store extra fat while dieting (the body preparing for the next deprivation), which can easily explain weight gain over time.[4] Willpower alone won't cut it. While we may be able to control what we eat and drink, we are not in conscious control of how our bodies use energy.[5] Genetic variations, medications, medical conditions, gut microbial composition and stress all alter energy (calorie) utilization.[5] And again, **we can't control these things**!

<u>Dieting interferes with weight regulation in the following ways:</u>[4]

- o Slows the rate at which your body burns calories
- o Causes craving of high-fat foods
- o Increases appetite
- o Reduces energy level

o Lowers body temperature, causing you to use less energy and feel cold
o Increases fat-storage enzymes and decreases fat-release enzymes
o Reduces your ability to recognize hunger and fullness
o Reduces total amount of muscle tissue (which burns more calories than fat)
o Increases fat-storage enzymes and decreases fat-release enzymes

More proof that you didn't fail the diet, the diet failed you.[4]

You can minimize the damage by swearing off diets once and for all. We do understand that you may be wanting weight loss, and that's not what sets you up for failure, it's the dieting (food restriction) that's detrimental. We'll explain how weight can be normalized healthfully with the right mindset.

So what is the key?

The key is eating according to your body's appetite and cues without concern about your weight. We know this may sound impossible, but stick with us. This strategy does result in the body regulating itself and, therefore, weight stability*—no drastic measures needed. In the following pages, we will walk you through tools that we've seen help our patients, friends, colleagues and ourselves!

---

* Weight stability means lack of significant fluctuation in weight over time. Adults have a genetically determined "set point"—a healthy weight range your body tries to maintain. However, it's important to note that one's setpoint may not be in line with is considered "ideal" (by oneself or the dreaded BMI scale).[4]

How to use this book

What we are suggesting is likely NEW to you. It's not a "quick fix." It may ultimately be the OPPOSITE of what you've been doing. But it's time to try something new. And it is absolutely necessary if you want ultimate freedom from the ever-present burden food has become. Freedom to live life more fully and be able to focus on what really matters in your life. Through our personal and professional experiences, we have witnessed and helped others struggling in many of the same ways you may be.

We have *not* invented a program or brand-new concepts, rather we have compiled tools and strategies from our own experiences and other leaders in the field. We put them together in a readable and applicable way to help you **make peace with food so you can end the war with your body!†**

---

† This book is not recommended if you are engaging in eating disorder behaviors such as vomiting, use of laxatives, over-exercise, etc. Working with a nutritionist and therapist who specialize in eating disorders is recommended. Please visit https://www.psychologytoday.com to find treatment in your area.

FREE TO BE TOOLS

Waving the White Flag

Tools for forming a lasting truce with yourself

This section will give you tools to help you learn about yourself and your motivations. After each tool is described in this section, you will find "action ■━━▷ items" designated by a pencil that will guide you in learning about yourself in regard to that specific area. _We recommended designating a special notebook or online document to use as you go through the action items._

After the tool section, there is a worksheet. We suggest the worksheet be used as daily guide to help you practice the different tools reviewed in the section that are most applicable to you and your relationship with food and your body. We expect certain tools to resonate with you more than others, given that these are not "rules" or a step-by-step guide. The tools that are the most helpful will be based on your own history and current experiences. There are affirmations sprinkled throughout which can be used at any time. One idea is to have a go-to list of affirmations that appeal to you and pick one to focus on each day.

First things first - where are you now?

▪️▬▶ Identify how the DIET MENTALITY currently impacts your thinking.

How much of your life have you spent on a diet? Before you picked up this book, were you actively on a diet, contemplating a diet, "off the wagon" or somewhere between?

▪️▬▶ How much time are you spending thinking about food?

What would you love to be doing instead? Examples: writing, learning a new skill, focusing on family relationships, reconnecting with friends, etc.

▪️▬▶ How have your feelings about your body or food held you back?

What are you NOT doing that you want to do? Examples: dating, spending time with friends or family, traveling, etc.

1

FREE TO BE TOOL

Change Your Goals

We know—cue the eye roll—but keep reading! Make your goal to improve health and achieve body acceptance, neutrality, respect rather than solely focusing on weight loss. We are NOT ignoring the fact that you want weight normalization, we are providing recommended tools to lead you there. However, the reality is that weight does not determine health. Health is both physical and emotional and is influenced by many factors including stress level, quality of sleep, genetics and relationships. If we focus only on weight, our focus is not in trying to <u>avoid</u> behaviors instead of <u>adding</u> positive habits and enjoyment. **A fixation on weight alone neglects many factors that contribute to our overall well-being, and consequently takes us away from addressing factors that maintain excess weight.**

In addition, it is well known that people can be fit and fat. Physical activity attenuates the risk of metabolic and cardiovascular diseases associated with excess weight. Consider the following evidence that larger body size does not equal poor health:

- o A review of health data (blood pressure, cholesterol, blood sugar, and a CRP, a marker of inflammation) in 40,420 adults revealed that nearly half of those considered overweight by BMI standards and 29% of those considered obese were metabolically healthy. However, <u>over 30% of normal weight individuals were cardiometabolically unhealthy.</u>[6]
- o In >11,000 adults followed for 7 years, only those who were inactive had a significantly increased risk of all-cause mortality independent of weight status.[7]
- o In a cohort-based study of 7,438 Australian women and 6,053 men aged 71–79, being overweight conferred the lowest risk of death within 10 years compared with being obese or having normal weight.[8]

Diet culture would have us default to a superficial body "goal," such as being a certain size or weight, which may or may not be realistic or sustainable. (See Tool 2 for more on body image). This "default" message was illustrated recently when I (SA) walked into a new fitness facility. Part of the intake process was being asked: What is your goal? My thoughts immediately went to what I felt I was **expected** to say. Be more toned? Lose inches or a certain number of pounds? It's unfortunate that my REAL goals, to challenge myself and feel well, didn't come to me right away.

This leads us to the elephant in the room—our influences. If you are committed to changing your goal to FEELING WELL mentally and physically, it's important to minimize the visuals that contribute to negative body image. More specifically, we suggest UNFOLLOWING social media accounts that promote diet or weight loss and trigger negative thoughts (you know the hashtags). If you've ever felt down after comparing your body to others, you know how unproductive and unnecessary this is.

▪▆▆▷ What are your goals regarding body image?

Examples: stop the negative self-talk about a particular part of your body, feel more confident in public, romantic relationship or workplace.

▪▆▆▷ What are your physical health goals?

Examples: reduce or eliminate the need for diabetes or blood pressure medication, have more energy, be able to play with your children/grandchildren, complete a 5K, practice yoga or a martial art.

▪▆▆▷ What has your body done for you?

Examples: carries you outdoors to walk your dog and breathe fresh air, creates and allows you to care for human being(s), allows you to experience things you enjoy (listen to music, enjoy the beach, examples with all senses). *Refer to this list when having negative body thoughts.

▪▆▆▷ List any influences (social media or otherwise) that leave you feeling depleted or negative about yourself.

What might you replace those influences with? See resource section for examples of more positive social media.

▪▆▆▷ Practice affirmations for positive reinforcement:
- I am thankful for what my body can do
- I refuse to shame or hate my body
- My body is ok right now, the way it is
- I am strong in body and mind and can overcome challenge

2

FREE TO BE TOOL

Focus on Values, Not your Appearance

One of the main keys to weight normalization is to focus on what matters (not the shape of your body!). By focusing on what really matters in your life, it will help to diffuse the inaccurate message that our power and happiness come from our bodies. Cultural messages and marketing lead us to believe that our appearance strongly relates to our happiness. This is simply not true. If you look at empirically validated studies about happiness and life satisfaction, the results consistently show that happy people have strong connections with other people and their communities.[9] Physical attractiveness is *not* noted as a strong contributing factor to happiness.

When you feel pulled to focus on your body, remind yourself that body shapes and sizes considered to be desirable are completely arbitrary. Throughout history and across cultures, completely different shapes and sizes have been considered attractive. Until more recently, even in Westernized cultures, what was considered to be attractive was related more to health than a specific body shape or size. For example, body fat is needed to maintain reproductive health, so it makes sense that what was considered to be attractive was NOT extreme thinness. Unrealistic and inappropriate cultural expectations about the way you should look go against our own biology.

> Body shapes and sizes considered to be desirable are completely arbitrary.

If you want to like and treat your body well, most people think you first must like your appearance. However, even if you are unhappy with your appearance, you can still have a positive body image. This is because positive body image is not contingent on appearance, it's created by respecting and accepting your body. If you focus on things like your personality and the physical strength of your body—truly looking beyond your appearance—that focus allows positive body image to develop. Said in a different way, positive body image is about appreciating your true self (your internal attributes) and the functionality of your body, it's not about feeling attractive or being a certain weight, size or shape.

We hear people say that if they lose weight or look a different way then certain opportunities or experiences will become available to them. However, there are *completely* different cultural (e.g., body-shape, age, race, etc.) perceptions of what is considered attractive or unattractive, as well as documented stereotypes that individuals hold related to weight and attractiveness (e.g., the physical attractiveness stereotype is assuming that people who are physically attractive also have other socially desirable personality traits). Therefore, the only realistic anecdote to all these mixed messages and stereotypes is to <u>stay true to what you want for yourself</u> and focus on your health, not your appearance.

Simply put, the more you are living a life that is in line with what you want, the easier it is to view food as just food and your body for what it is, a vessel to honor since it allows us to pursue our true values.

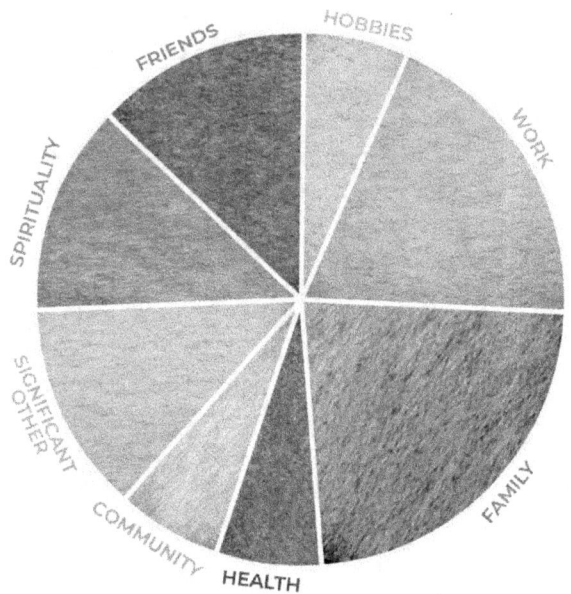

What aspects of your life mean the most and deserve your love and attention? (Examples of values above adapted from *Valued Living Questionnaire* by Kelly Wilson & Groom)

> ▶ List the things that mean the most to you. What makes life worth living?

> ▶ List 3 things you want to spend MORE time doing and 3 things you want to spend LESS time doing.

> ▶ Identify what is stopping you from doing what you truly want so you can begin working around those barriers.

3

FREE TO BE TOOL

Learn about Your Relationship with Food

We want you to be a curious observer about your relationship with food. We suggest you think of it as observing, rather than **judging or criticizing** your eating habits. When you are inquisitive about what and how you eat, it allows you to see how you may be eating out of habit, when you're tired, stressed, angry or when you're not liking your body.

In my clinical practice (AH), I often hear how people want to eat when they are experiencing body shame. This may seem counterintuitive, but it actually makes sense because when you're beating yourself up, you need to feel better! Food is so tricky because it DOES make us feel better momentarily. The feel-good chemicals like serotonin and dopamine surge when food hits our taste-buds. Unfortunately, that pleasurable surge only creates a <u>temporary</u> break or mood boost. Often, people say they feel even worse after eating when they weren't hungry. Therefore, we encourage you to study yourself before and after you eat and learn to nurture your true needs instead of eating as a way to self soothe after feeling beat up.

Try to slow down and ask yourself the following questions before you eat:

1. Am I hungry? (see hunger/fullness scale in worksheet)
2. What am I feeling? (go to the emotion list if you can't identify)
3. Do I want to eat to fill another need?
4. What food would nourish me physically right now?

Don't be afraid of hunger. It is a natural body signal that should be welcomed. When not attended to, hunger results in overeating even for the most intuitive eater.

It is very important to decide not to feel guilty about whatever you're going to eat before eating. It is extremely liberating to realize that nothing bad happens if you don't beat yourself up. In fact, something good happens—you actually enjoy the food! Then notice how your BODY feels. Feel free to write it down. If you are someone who often feels guilt related to food, this exercise is an absolute must and a HUGE step in the direction of peace with food. Removing the guilt factor is essential for being able to tune into physical body cues.[4,10] Committing to letting go of food-related guilt no matter what was the number one thing that helped me (SA) move past preoccupation with food and weight.

> Removing the guilt factor is essential for being able to tune into physical body cues.[4,10]

FREE TO BE TOOL

When you Want to Eat, but you're NOT Hungry

As we discussed previously, when you want to eat but know you're not hungry, the food is code for something else that you are currently needing. Take the pressure off by taking a deep breath, slow down and try to focus on your true need. When you aren't hungry but want to eat, this is often when the diet mentality kicks in. Reject the "now or never" and "all or nothing" ways of thinking that are typically components of diets. When we recognize that we can enjoy things in moderation <u>every day</u>, that's when food loses its power over us. Freedom comes from realizing that you don't have to eat everything because there's always tomorrow, and there's always more food. Recognize abundance. Depending on your upbringing, food may or may not have been readily available (either due to lack of food or restriction of food). These feelings related to food certainly carry over into adulthood and can lead to overeating. It may take time to reassure yourself that you CAN have the food in question, and it WILL be available when you want it, but this is another critical step in achieving independence from feeling controlled by food.[11] For some, it is helpful to carry snacks to reiterate the awareness of abundance.[11]

Other helpful things to remind yourself:

○ Eating doesn't meet our true emotional needs; it's only a temporary boost of feel-good chemicals

○ When you're hyper-focused on your body, review your True Values List (worksheet at the end of book)

○ Remember that food will be more enjoyable to eat when you are hungry

○ Identify the diet messages coming from yourself or others and ignore them (e.g. "Eat it all now, even if you aren't hungry, and start the diet tomorrow")

○ Sometimes you just really want the food. If this is the case, **eat and enjoy it without regret!**

▸ Reflect on a typical week and notice your patterns without judgement. Are there certain parts of the day where you find yourself wanting to eat?

Many people find themselves grazing or wanting to eat more in the evening if they <u>have not eaten enough during the day</u>. In this case, making a point to eat more during the day can be the fix. Soon, you will be hungrier during the day and you will naturally eat less later in the day, when your metabolic processes are less efficient.[12]

▸ List your triggers for eating too much or feeling out of control while eating. Examples: time of day, getting TOO hungry, or stressful daily events.

▸ How (in addition to eating) could you address those "trigger" feelings?

▸ Practice affirmation for positive reinforcement:
  – Food will not fulfill my true feelings/needs

24

Mindful eating exercise

Mindful eating means paying attention to sensory information while eating. It involves slowing down and avoiding distractions (eating while doing **nothing** else)! Mindful eating helps you tune into your body, enjoy food and improve your relationship with food. *

Here is a sample mindful eating exercise:

o Choose a small food like a raisin or piece of chocolate.
o Observe the food and notice its shape, texture and smell.
o What are thoughts you have regarding the food? (Like/dislike, judgements)
o How is the food grown or made?
o Bring the food to your mouth and hold it there for at least 10 seconds.
o Notice texture, how it feels.
o Take time to chew without swallowing, noticing any change in taste and feeling of the food in your mouth.
o When you feel ready to swallow, bring awareness to the sensation.
o Notice what is left of the food as you swallow.
o Notice how your body feels after completing this exercise.

The expectation is not for you to eat every bite of every meal with this much awareness, but to practice being MORE aware while eating.

---

* Lynn Rossy's book (listed in resources) is an excellent comprehensive guide for mindful eating.

5

FREE TO BE TOOL

Studying Yourself after you Eat

After you eat is the perfect time to gather more data about your relationship with food. This step involves many of the tools previously listed in order to help continue to flush out how you meet your needs and what you may continue to need moving forward. This may seem redundant but it's an important step in learning about how you personally use food. After you eat, ask yourself:

1. Did I eat because I was hungry? It's ok either way—this is a learning process. If no, then eating was soothing another need (bored, tired, etc.). That's ok too! Try not to judge yourself for trying to meet your needs. Meeting our needs is a healthy thing. The ultimate goal is to nurture our true needs.
2. What need was I trying to fill? Avoid judgment and instead use this as a learning experience. Feeling shame typically only leads to more eating!
3. How does my body feel now? If we can tune in and listen, our bodies tend to "tell" us what they want.

How does my body feel after eating?

- o Bloated
- o Light
- o Energized
- o Too full
- o Heavy
- o Shaky

- o Upset stomach
- o Foggy
- o Clear-headed
- o Gassy
- o Tired

- o Nauseated
- o Distended
- o Crampy
- o Comfortable

When focusing on how your body physically feels, you may be inclined to also feel guilty about what you did or didn't eat. We've already touched on the counterproductive nature of guilt. A recent study showed that participants who felt guilt instead of celebration about eating chocolate cake were less successful in maintaining their weight over an 18-month period.[13] This makes sense if you think about how when we feel bad about something, we are motivated to feel better. What is a quick way to feel better? Eating! Therefore, if you don't feel bad about what you've done (because you haven't done anything wrong!), you aren't setting yourself up to continue this exhausting cycle:

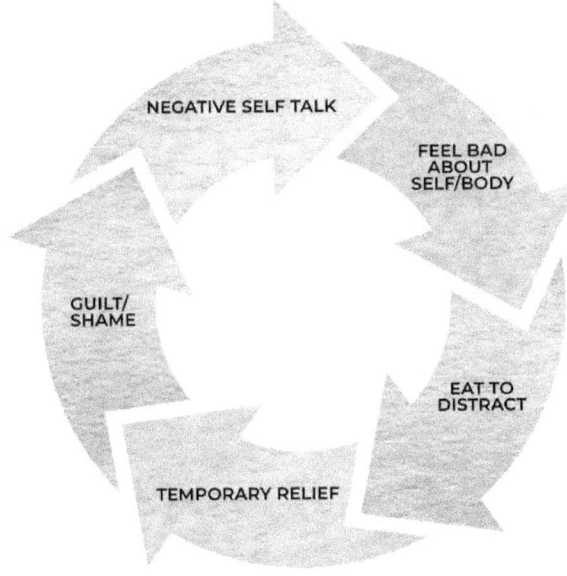

If you ate when you weren't hungry, in addition to trying to understand the trigger, we encourage you to eat again when you feel hungry. Resuming a normal routine helps get you metabolically back on track and prevent the guilt and non-hunger eating cycle discussed above. It is important NOT to restrict food, as this will only further propagate the cycle.

The goal is a cycle of eating that looks more like this:

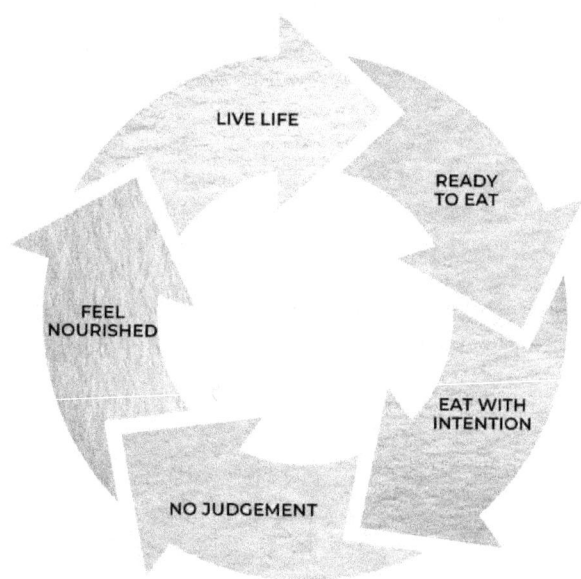

6

FREE TO BE TOOL

Prioritize Self-Care

Self-care is anything you do to be good to yourself. It is essential for our physical, emotional and mental well-being. When learning to let go of diets, self-care keeps us on the right path by reinforcing positive feelings toward ourselves and helping us cope with negative emotions. Self-care is an essential part of the journey toward wellness, not a reward or luxury.

You've probably heard the saying that you have to take care of yourself before you can take care of others. You don't have energy for others without caring for yourself first. Self-care is the opposite of selfishness! It BENEFITS others when we take care of ourselves. When we are busy and overwhelmed it's easy to neglect ourselves, but this leads to issues like burnout, illness, unhappiness and the inability to tend to and support others. Think about how you're already practicing self-care. Most ways aren't indulgent. You brush your teeth, drink water, rejuvenate yourself with sleep, go to the dentist, connect with friends, and hopefully laugh and smile. Recognize these things for what they are, ways you take care of yourself!

▮▬▷ List what self-care things you already do. List things you really enjoy and make a plan to do them more often.

What is fun and makes you feel good? Examples: reading, taking a bath, going to a movie, listening to music, getting a massage, spending time with loved ones, playing, expressing your creativity (painting, pottery, scrapbooking, crafts).

▮▬▷ List self-care things you *aren't* doing that you'd find nurturing.

Components of self-care:

- o Stress management
- o Movement
- o Sleep
- o Nourishment

Stress management

Stress is a necessary function of life. It's the activation of the sympathetic nervous system in response to a demand or threat. In its most useful forms, stress motivates you to prepare for a task or helps protect you from danger. Everyone experiences stress, most often in the form of *routine* stress, like the demands of work, school and family. On the other hand, *acute* stress is a sudden negative change like job loss, illness or an accident.

When stress becomes chronic, the immune system becomes suppressed and people often experience physical symptoms like low energy, headaches, digestive trouble, difficulty sleeping and more. In addition, too much stress clouds our ability to recognize priorities and makes our self-care goals seem insignificant. We can't get RID of stress but learning how to manage it is the first step in any self-improvement process.

We can't get RID of stress but learning how to manage it is the first step in any self-improvement process.

What's causing you the most stress? Sometimes it's an unhealthy relationship or a dreaded job. These are parts of your life that can be altered, though no one said it would be easy. Other times, the only thing we can change is our <u>response</u> to the stress. We can always control that part—how we view and use the obstacle—by making a conscious choice to do so. We can also choose to limit the factors in our lives that are consistently associated with negative feelings. An example of this that we've already touched on would be unfollowing social media accounts that may be adding to negative feelings about oneself or unrealistic self-comparisons. We can choose to invest in nurturing relationships and friendships instead.

◀▬▷ What positive actions help you release stress?

Examples: talking with your support system, journaling, movement, breathing exercises, meditation or a combination of things. If you're unsure, try some of these.

◀▬▷ List your body's signs of increased stress.

Examples: headache, neck pain, fatigue, gastrointestinal distress, moodiness or behavior changes, etc.

Externalize and sit with It

When feeling particularly stressed or anxious, try setting a timer and allowing yourself to worry or let go of control for a set period of time (like 2-5 minutes). Allow the feeling to run its course and naturally diffuse. Observe the emotions being released. Example: for 5 minutes I am going to worry about X and then I'm going to let it go.

Mental release

◀▬▷ List stressors that you cannot control and then let them go.

◀▬▷ Practice affirmations for positive reinforcement.

- Where I am right now is exactly where I need to be

- I am at peace with what is, what was, and what will be

Movement

Our bodies were made to move. Movement should feel good, not like torture! We need to move to feel well, to <u>be able to do the things we want to do</u> and strengthen our body and mind. Movement is NOT to "earn" our food, compensate for what's already been eaten, or to lose weight.

When we focus on activity for weight loss purposes *only*:

o   We minimize the other benefits conferred like increased energy, decreased stress, improved cognitive function and better sleep, to name a few.
o   We forget to enjoy it.
o   Because we don't enjoy it and our "goal" isn't met, we don't stick with it.

Movement, anything from yoga to dancing to walking, can reduce cortisol levels (secreted by adrenal glands in response to stress) and increase endorphins (feel-good brain chemicals). Movement is also known to leave you feeling better about your body.

Focusing on movement for psychological and physical health benefits may be a major shift in thinking. Some in the fitness industry bank on using exercise as a way for you to literally "buy in" to the weight loss and body ideals, but YOU don't have to. The truth is less desirable than we all hoped...we'd have to be Olympic athletes for movement alone to result in significant weight loss. But we don't have to be Michael Phelps to glean some major benefits from physical activity.

<u>We suggest movement hedonism: being active because you want to</u> in order to relieve stress and gain energy, mental clarity, flexibility, strength, stamina, self-respect and even friends! This means avoiding calculating the number of calories burned or

forcing yourself to do an activity for a certain period of time. This does NOT mean you shouldn't work hard or have physical goals. Work hard for the right reasons—because it makes you feel good and strong and proud.

Work hard for the right reasons—because it makes you feel good and strong and proud.

It's important to note that you don't have to have a strict plan in place for directed activity. Just find ways to move more and do it often, whether it be walking over lunch or doing some quick moves when you have a few minutes. Doing an activity outside results in even more mood-boosting effects.

You don't have to be a researcher to know that people tend to retain habits they enjoy. Throughout this book we are suggesting ADDING enjoyment to your life (enjoying food, enjoying movement) and taking away the strict rules that set us up for failure.

✎➤ List what activities feel best for YOUR body (during or after).

What movements make you feel most energized or relaxed? Examples: walking, dancing, swimming, jogging, stretching, boxing, etc.). If moving is difficult or painful, are there more gentle movements you could consider (swimming, yoga, Tai Chi)?

✎➤ What is a new activity you could try or something you used to enjoy that you could pick back up? Zumba, yoga, cycling, swimming?

Sleep

The relationship between lack of adequate sleep and weight gain is well established.[14,15] One-third of Americans report getting less than the recommended 7+ hours of sleep per night.[16] Too little sleep increases the hunger hormone (ghrelin) and decreases the satiety hormone (leptin). All of our cells operate on a circadian clock, and offsetting this by not sleeping enough during the night results in decreased immune function and increased inflammation, risk of type 2 diabetes, heart disease and depression. A simplified way to think about this is to remember that we fuel our bodies with food and sleep. If one is off, it typically throws the other off. To stay alert, our bodies adapt to physiologically crave food when we are tired. Therefore, when we have a normal sleep cycle, we're setting ourselves up to be more in tune with our system's true needs related to fuel and rest.

Many people find that there is a particular time of day when they are most productive. Just like with food, we're _not_ suggesting that everyone be on the same schedule or adhere to strict sleep rules. Instead, be mindful of how well and how much you're sleeping and make sleep a priority.

▐▆▅▅▆➤ List things that are keeping you awake.

Examples: stress, television, anxious thoughts, work, etc.

▐▆▅▅▆➤ What could you do to prioritize sleep?

Is there a different time of day you could attend to things listed in action item above? If worry is more prevalent at night, could you try going to bed earlier or try a calming affirmation or meditation app?

Nutrition

This is a difficult topic for anyone with a history of frequent dieting, preoccupation with food, or strict "food rules." Let's start with a fact check:

True: Our bodies need nourishment to survive and thrive.

False: We need to avoid certain foods in order to be healthy.

True: Some foods are more nutrient dense than others.

False: Eating foods considered "unhealthy" will make you "unhealthy."

True: We should be aware of what we eat.

False: We need to strictly plan and control what we eat.

As is illustrated above, the short answer to "what to eat" is: eat what makes you feel well and conveys respect for your body. But it takes some practice listening to our bodies and not judging what we're eating to get there. Jump into nutrition information too early in your process, and it can turn into another diet. We recommend NOT looking at nutrition labels to start with. The calorie count, grams of fat, carbohydrates or sugar don't matter as much as: 1) Are you hungry? 2) Do you want the food? 3) How do you feel physically after eating?

Eventually, when you can see a food or nutrition label without judging it as "good or bad" and eat any food without experiencing guilt, it may be more reasonable to be a curious observer of nutrition facts.[10] In the end, nobody knows your body better than you, so have some healthy skepticism for anyone "telling" you what to eat. Let any feelings of judgement pass, as too many people are still clouded by the old (tried and NOT true) diet mentality.

It is also important to note that you don't have to have a "perfect" diet to be healthy. One particular food isn't going to clog your arteries or cause diabetes just because it's not dense in nutrients. It's the balance over time that matters. Likely more important than WHAT you're eating is HOW you're feeling about it and whether you ENJOY it, because as we've mentioned, the negative impact of stress surrounding eating may very well be worse for you than any food in question.

Likely more important than WHAT you're eating is HOW you're feeling about it and whether you ENJOY it.

FREE TO BE TOOL

Practice Self-Compassion

The way we form new habits is through repetition. Practicing the same thought patterns and behaviors creates new neural pathways that help a new habit "stick." Practice taking it easy on yourself. In a study of 435 women in the US, self-compassion was associated with a decrease in disordered eating and decreased influence of thinness-related pressures.[17]

Here are final suggestions that may be useful to implement as you move through the tools we've provided.

1. Stop beating yourself up: if the goal is body-acceptance versus weight loss, then you won't need the behaviors that comfort you when you are preoccupied with body dissatisfaction or other negative emotions. We consistently see that the people who focus on health instead of beating themselves up end up NOT managing emotions with food. This is KEY!

2. Simply say STOP! out loud when you're thinking negative or judgmental thoughts about what you've eaten. Or picture a big red stop sign.

3. Be a friend to yourself. Don't say things to yourself that you wouldn't say to someone you dearly love and respect. It may be helpful to externalize any self-criticism to a trusted friend. Hearing the criticism out loud and getting support can help you tap into self-compassion and diffuse the negative (and often irrational!) self-criticism.

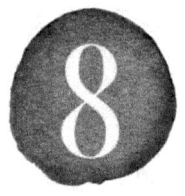

FREE TO BE TOOL

Expectations for the Process

By practicing the tools that are applicable to your own life—whether focusing more on your values or true emotional needs—we ultimately want you to experience a sense of freedom. We understand that you want this to happen quickly, but it's important to remember that it will take time to undo a lifetime of diet-centered thoughts and goals. Working through the tools in this book will take time and practice.

This process will look different for everyone, given our unique life experiences and genetics. Don't expect a speedy linear path; you will likely cycle back and forth through different tools, and your answers to the action items or goals may evolve over time.

There may be times when you feel like you're making significant progress, but then start to regress into old habits or ways of thinking. It's ok! **If you find yourself in a "setback," remember that it's normal and you're still way ahead of where you started.** You won't be perfect. You may eat too much food, and your body may feel less than ideal. It's usually not about the food. But you'll take a deep breath and know nothing terrible will happen. You'll shake it off and reset your mind and NOT feel guilty or shameful. You're still in it. You're NOT back where you started. You know too much now.

You know too much now.

In addition to patience, we should also have realistic expectations. It would be unfair to ourselves to believe that our bodies should stay the same over our lifespan. Even if we could magically maintain our weight, things like our skin texture and elasticity (think wrinkles and cellulite) will change due to natural hormonal shifts related to the unstoppable aging process. Therefore, our bodies SHOULD look different at ages 20, 30, 40, 50, etc. Given that we cannot stop aging, just like with body image and weight, we need to focus on our true values and health in order not to feel a sense of constant discontent that would come from denying a completely natural human process.

We wrote this book to be a concise and readable resource that can be easily integrated and revisited in your day-to-day life. <u>With time and practice, we are confident you can feel at ease around food and at peace in your own body. Practice makes progress.</u>

➤ List three goals that are important to you related to food, diet, or body-image.

Examples: make conscious food choices without guilt, feel comfortable at family gatherings, reintroduce previously "off limits" foods, learn to let go of negative self-talk.

Examples of long-term goals:

- o   Feel comfortable around food
- o   Feel comfortable in body
- o   Feel free to think about other things

- ○ Feel free to pursue a passion
- ○ Refuse to participate in body bashing and self-deprecation
- ○ Refuse to buy into diet culture myths and fads like diets or medication

Closing thoughts

Mindset

Mindset is the single most powerful determining factor of your success.

Make a commitment to reframe your mindset in four steps:

1. Give yourself permission to stop participating in anything that promotes dieting or weight loss
2. Observe yourself and learn about yourself from these observations
3. Reframe your thoughts to foster self-appreciation and self-trust
4. Make meaningful, lasting habit changes that you enjoy and reinforce these with positive influences

Have you ever felt good about yourself after waking up in the morning only to have those feelings demolished by the number on the scale? Did ANYTHING about your body actually change from the time before you stepped on the scale until you saw the number? Not physically of course, only your mind changed. How could you have prevented this? Either A) deciding not to weigh yourself or B) deciding ahead of time that what the number says will not negatively affect you. That internal dialogue has a direct effect on your emotions and behavior. Work on changing your mindset to change your behavior.

▮▬▶What are some reasons you are proud of yourself?

Think of a recent time when a different mindset would've changed everything.

■➡️ Practice affirmations for positive
reinforcement:
- Only I determine my path today. My success begins in my mind.
- I am worthy of all good things.
- I will treat myself with love and respect.

Our mind is the only thing we truly have total control over. That's why it's so important to make some mindset adjustments and promise that:

- I can and will treat myself with kindness and respect
- I am more than the numbers that "define" me or the food that I ate
- I am strong and capable and pretty badass for a lot of reasons

I am strong and capable and pretty badass for a lot of reasons.

FOOD PEACE WORKSHEET

Remember that these are tools that you'll cycle through when you're wanting to eat when not hungry and/or you're not liking your body. There are no wrong or right rules or steps!

I. When you are physically hungry: eat!

Focus on what tastes good to you and what your system would benefit from and honor your system's need to fuel and nourish the body and mind. Plate your food and while you're eating, enjoy texture, taste, etc. After eating realistic portion for your body's needs, PAUSE and NOTICE. Slowing down and checking in with yourself at this moment is key in order to get your true needs met! If you feel you don't know when you're hungry, see the Resource Section about the Hunger Experiment.

Hunger/Fullness Scale

1	Empty/too hungry - irritable, shaky, lack of concentration
2	Hungry - mild gnawing or growling feeling in stomach, ready to eat, thinking of food
3	Neutral - not hungry or full
4	Full - feel food in stomach, satisfied
5	Too full - uncomfortable, stuffed, sick

2. Still wanting to eat when not hungry? Identify what you're really feeling.

Emotions! Emotions! Emotions! Wanting to eat is code for another need. Accept our needs! What are you really feeling?

List YOUR emotions(s) here:

_____

_____

_____

_____

_____

_____

Shame	Angry	Depressed	Drained
Guilty	Confused	Exhausted	Worthless
Resentment	Directionless	Rejected	Helpless
Dejected	Trapped	Empty	Defeated
Grief	Overwhelmed	Disappointed	Offended
Hopeless	Jealous	Inadequate	Controlled
Lonely	Smothered	Dismissed	Panicky
Irritable	Agitated	Judged	Terrified
Scared	Embarrassed	Unappreciated	Frantic
Worried	Drained	Disillusioned	
Nervous	Hurt	Alienated	

3. Meeting the need related to feeling

Once emotion(s) are identified, identify behaviors that will actually nurture the true need vs. meeting the need with food.

Examples of self-care to cope with emotional needs:

1. I am mad about work, so I'm going to go on a walk to release tension

2. I am feeling lonely, so I'm going to call a friend

3. I feel anxious, I will externalize my fears in my journal

Self-Care Options:

1. Getting out of your head by <u>distraction</u>. Examples: watching funny TV, hanging with friends, reading.
2. <u>Talking</u> it out with your support system. Examples: connecting with family, friend, spiritual advisor, therapist, or support group via email, text, call, or meeting up.
3. <u>Nurturing physical/emotional needs</u>: Examples: sleep, externalizing emotions in a journal, physical movement, quiet time alone, unplugging from technology.
4. <u>Reframing thoughts</u>: Examples: recognizing that emotions are feelings not facts, ask yourself if there's another way of looking at a situation, understand that feelings are malleable by trying to find the silver lining.

List how you can meet emotional need:

_____

_____

_____

_____

_____

_____

4. If you're not liking your body and want to eat: focus on true values

The natural by-product of living your life within you own values system means that and body image will take a back-seat to our true priorities. Subsequently we will fuel and nourish our bodies based on system's needs, not our emotional needs.

List of Values[18] (List is meant to generate self-focus, not meant to imply that one should value all areas):

1. Spirituality (e.g., communicating with nature, participation with organized religion)
2. Leisure hobbies (animals, sports, nature, etc.)
3. Aesthetics (art, music, literature, etc.)
4. Relation with romantic partner
5. Relations with friends
6. Community involvement (e.g., political, charity, caring for environment, etc.)
7. Work or career
8. Family (other than romantic partner and parenting)
9. Physical health (values related to sleep, movement, diet, etc.)

True Values:

_____

_____

_____

_____

_____

_____

5: Still thinking about appearance or weight? Shift focus to internal and physical attributes (true self focus)

Debunk the myths! Our body is NOT our value or source of happiness, despite what we've been repeatedly told from uncountable sources. If we focus on what truly matters in life, we will be free to focus on meeting our true needs and not turning to food to try to fill us up.

State AFFIRMATION: <u>My worth is not my body. Eating when I don't like my body will not bring me the peace I'm looking for. Meeting my true needs is my goal.</u>

Honoring True Self by listing what you like about yourself that is not related to your body or appearance. Examples; kind, funny, hard-worker, creative, etc.

I like that I am:

_____

_____

_____

_____

_____

_____

FAQs and Resources

This last section includes many commonly asked questions as well as additional resources to help support you!

1. What if I don't know when I'm hungry? The Hunger Experiment

We see patients who have lost touch with the way hunger feels or what their body may be needing. Similarly, we've consistently observed that the more shame people feel about their bodies, the more DISCONNECTED they are from their physical needs. It seems that the more you don't like your body, the more you ignore its cues. The goal is to reconnect with what your system needs and to nurture those needs!

If you are not sure you recognize hunger and satiety signals, you may try another experiment—waiting longer to eat breakfast or lunch to notice how your body tells you you're hungry. It is absolutely true that skipping meals can lead to overeating later. What we are suggesting is just holding off on a meal, <u>not</u> skipping it all together. Does your stomach growl, feel empty? Does the sensation go away after several minutes, then return? Once you've paid attention to this for 30-60 minutes, eat a meal mindfully.

2. What is an Ideal Eating Plan?

Just as the tools that work for you may not be the same ones that work for everyone, what works best for YOU and your sister/neighbor/cousin may be different. Actual food and frequency are individual—some people function better on 3 meals per day, some with several smaller meals. Real food eaten when hungry, enjoyed, nourishes you, and makes your body feel good would be ideal. But for the love of all things holy, make sure it is food you ENJOY! THIS has been a key piece missing from your diet-life until this point. This is not to suggest that every meal should be gourmet. It's about WHY you're choosing that food—to nourish and take care of yourself, to feel well and live longer.

We decided NOT to include factual nutrition information primarily because it is probable that you have some work to do in changing your mindset regarding eating before thinking about nutrition and functionality of food. Discussing nutrition too soon can create another set of rules (diet mentality). Additionally, it is likely that you pretty much know what foods are nutrient dense.

3. I'm scared that I will gain weight during this process. How do I handle my fears?

As you're going through this process, it's absolutely normal if you feel a spike in anxiety or body dissatisfaction. This is because anxiety is often triggered by the unknown, and it's impossible to know whether someone will gain or lose some weight during this process, especially if weight has been suppressed by dieting. This process requires you to lean into the unknown and trust that as you fuel your system as it needs, your body *can* be trusted to recalibrate to its set-point. Your set-point is the biologically determined weight your body prefers for optimal function.

When anxiety is triggered, gently remind yourself to breathe, focus on your true values related to health, and practice self-care related to your anxiety. Ideas include: go for a walk, meditate, read a calming message/passage/affirmation, reach out for support (such as the Free To Be Facebook page). Be comforted by the fact that individuals who eat intuitively do eventually have normalized weight, healthy body image, and that there are no documented adverse effects for any of the tools in this book. Ride the wave of uncertainty and your body and mind will thank you later.

4. What if I have certain allergy or medical issues?

If you have diet restrictions for medical reasons—celiac disease, food sensitivities, diabetes, heart disease, etc., how you frame your choices and your system's dietary needs is key. For example, the outlook would ideally be one of "I want to do this for my body" instead of "I have to do this because my doctor said so." Change your mindset to the WHY (thinking of it as a kind-to-body choice instead of restriction). Seek to understand the disease process and make a conscious decision based on BOTH what you want and what is best for you. The two don't have to be mutually exclusive, though it may take trying <u>new foods or different preparation methods</u> to maximize enjoyment. You are ultimately in charge of your thoughts and actions.

From a gastrointestinal functional standpoint, we do know that people can have dietary intolerances without being a named "disease." During the process of paying more attention to your body, you may notice that certain foods aren't well tolerated. First, try to make sure that the symptoms experienced are in the ABSENCE of a negative feeling toward the food. We know that being <u>fearful or anxious</u> (about ingestion of a food) can cause real symptoms!

Secondly, it is important to frame your choice regarding whether or not to eat the food around how it makes you feel rather than perceived positive or negative effect on weight or appearance. Example: a patient who knows that eating dairy causes abdominal cramping, bloating and diarrhea. He or she knows what will happen and may decide whether or not to eat a food containing dairy.

5. Is it ever ok to eat when I'm not hungry?

Yes. Everyone does it from time to time when something sounds good, something special is available, or for practical reasons. Maybe you're at a gathering or restaurant and not able to identify a need not being met. Or maybe you just want it! It's ok. Recognize the situation for what it is (e.g. "I want chocolate!"), make a conscious decision to eat it, enjoy the food, and move on. Without restricting food, labeling food as "good" or "bad," or feeling guilty after eating any food, you will find that intense cravings or desire to overeat dissipate.[4,10]

Because you are getting in touch with body cues and usually eating when hungry, eating when not hungry in this instance will not result in any sort of set-back. Nothing bad is going to happen. <u>Habits</u> are what matter most.

6. Do I have to choose the best food for my body all the time?

Absolutely not, that sounds boring! It's more about making a <u>conscious</u>, clear choice and being 100% ok with that choice. Do you really want the food? If so, ENJOY it then let it go...without regret or second-guessing. You will find that when you don't really desire the food and eat it anyway, it's not as satisfying.

7. I'm busy - how am I supposed to eat mindfully?

Make a point to start paying more attention during one meal per day. If mornings are rushed, could you take a few extra moments mid-day or in the evening? As you get more used to "tuning in," eat mindfully more regularly. This process is all about practicing making a point to *slow down* and *pay attention* as much as you can.

8. I am vegan for health and/or animal rights reasons. Are you saying it's wrong to be following a vegan diet?

No. There are plenty of people who avoid certain foods without a feeling of deprivation. However, we do suggest getting to a mentally healthy place with the suggestions listed in this book before attempting to cut any food out of your diet completely. How do you know when you're there? When you feel calm and at ease around food and fully lack judgement or guilt after eating.

9. I am finally on the path to creating a healthy relationship with food but am worried about my child who is showing signs of negative eating patterns. What should I do to help him/her?

We hope to be able to provide more guidance on this in another book. In the meantime, leading by example and being a positive role model regarding food and body image is the best place to start. The more we work on our personal issues, the less chance we have of transferring them. See recommendations listed below in our resource section. If your child is struggling with food issues on a daily basis, please seek out a qualified therapist in your area.

10. How do I deal with life issues that may be barriers to this process?

We recommend starting with self-care. While self-care is needed regardless of the type of stressors you're dealing with, care for yourself is even more vital when you are dealing with chronic stressors. Examples of these issues may be financial constraints, illness of self or family member, harmful relationships, child with an addiction, etc. Additional support like individual psychotherapy, family therapy, support groups, etc. may also be needed.

11. I'm thinking about having a bariatric procedure. How would surgery fit with this process?

If bariatric surgery has been recommended by a medical professional, you will have post-surgical medical and nutritional recommendations. The other tools recommended in this book are still very applicable to your journey. The post-surgical patients we see who have maintained long-term weight normalization typically have worked on their MINDSET in regard to commitment to developing a healthy relationship with food.

Resources

Professionals

Ashley Heintzelman, PhD. Licensed Psychologist and Eating Disorder Specialist https://drashleyheintzelman.com/

Katy Harvey, Certified Eating Disorder Registered Dietitian: https://katyharvey.net

Dr. Jennifer L. Gaudiani, MD, CEDS, FAED:

Eating Disorder Expert Physician: www.gaudianiclinic.com

Dr. Elissa Rosen, MD, CEDS: Eating Disorder Expert Physician: www.gaudianiclinic.com

Michelle Robin, DC: Founder and Chief Wellness Officer of Small Changes Big Shifts and Your Wellness Connection: https://www.yourwellnessconnection.com

Books that inspired our work

Intuitive Eating by E. Tribole and E. Resch, 2012

Health at Every Size by Linda Bacon, 2008

Body Respect by Linda Bacon and Lucy Aphramor, 2014

The Mindfulness-Based Eating Solution by Lynn Rossy, PhD, 2016

Body Kindness by Rebecca Scritchfield

Life Without ED by Jenni Schaefer and Thom Rutledge, 2003

Women, Food and God: An Unexpected Path to Almost Everything by Geneen Roth, 2011

The Gifts of Imperfection: Let Go of Who you Think You are Supposed to Be and Embrace Who You Are by Brene Brown, 2010

Positive Social Media Examples

Facebook

Free To Be Facebook group

Instagram

- Maryscupoftea
- Wellnessforthewin
- Damnthediets
- ditch_the_diet
- dietitiananna
- Thebodylovesociety
- Theintuitive_rd
- Ericaleonnutrition
- Annalutzrd
- yourpcosgirl

Podcasts

- Body Kindness
- Food Psych
- How to Love Your Body

Resources for Children

Child of Mine: Feeding with Love and Good Sense by Ellyn Satter

Ellyn Satter's website/newsletter - https://www.ellynsatterinstitute.org

Resources for Mindfulness and Stress Management

Center for mindful eating - https://www.thecenterformindfuleating.org/

Apps such as Insight Timer for meditation, relaxation.

The Obstacle is the Way by Ryan Holiday

Nutrition information (when ready, see p. 35)

https://www.hsph.harvard.edu/nutritionsource/

Finding a Pediatric or Adult Therapist

https://www.psychologytoday.com

Citations

[1] Wilke, Joy (2014, July 25). *Nearly half in U.S. remain worried about their weight, two-thirds of overweight Americans express concern about their current weight.* Retrieved from https://news.gallup.com/poll/174089/nearly-half-remain-worried-weight.aspx

[2] Reba-Harrelson, L., Von Holle, A., Hamer, R. M., Swann, R., Reyes, M. L., & Bulik, C. M. (2009). Patterns and prevalence of disordered eating and weight control behaviors in women ages 25-45. *Eating and weight disorders, 14*(4), 190-8. Retrieved from https://www.ncbi.nlm.nih.gov/pmc/articles/PMC3612547/

[3] Lenchewski, S. (2018). Food therapist. London: Sphere.

[4] Bacon, L. (2010). *Health at every size: the surprising truth about your weight.* Dallas, TX: BenBella Books.

[5] Bacon, L, & Aphramor, L. (2014). Body Respect: What Conventional Health Books Get Wrong, Leave out, and Just Plain Fail to Understand about Weight. BenBella Books.

[6] Tomiyama, A. J., Hunger, J. M., Nguyen-Cuu J., & Wells, C. (2016). Misclassification of cardiometabolic health when using body mass index categories in NHANES 2005–2012. *International Journal of Obesity, 40,* 883–886. DOI: 10.1038/ijo.2016.17

[7] Danke, S., Loenneke, J., & Loprinzi, D. (2016) Does the fat-but fit paradigm hold true for all-cause mortality when considering the duration of overweight/obesity? Analyzing the WATCH (Weight,

Activity and Time Contributes to Health) paradigm. *Preventive Medicine*, 83, 37-40. DOI: 10.1016/j.ypmed.2015.12.002

[8] Dobson, A, McLaughlin, D., Almeida, O., et al. (2012). Impact of behavioural risk factors on death within 10 years for women and men in their 70s: absolute risk charts. *BMC Public Health*, 12, 669. DOI: 10.1186/1471-2458-12-669

[9] Helliwell, J., Layard, R., & Sachs, J. (2018). World Happiness Report 2018. Retrieved from http://worldhappiness.report/ed/2018/

[10] Tribole, E. & Resc, E. (2012). *Intuitive eating - the revolutionary program that works.* (pp. 215) 215 New York, NY: St. Martin Griffin's.

[11] Harrison, C. (2018). Gentle Nutrition vs. Diet-Culture Nutrition with Heidi Schauster, Health At Every Size Nutrition Therapist. [podcast] Food Psych. Available at: http://foodpsych.libsyn.com/size/5/?search=Heidi+Schauster.

[12] Pawan, K.J., Challet, E., & Kalsbeek, A. (2015). Circadian rhythms in glucose and lipid metabolism in nocturnal and diurnal mammals. Molecular and Cellular Endocrinology, 418(1), 74-88. DOI: 10.1016/j.mce.2015.01.024

[13] Kuijer, R.G., & Boyce, J.A. (2014). Chocolate cake. Guilt or celebration? Associations with healthy eating attitudes, perceived behavioral control, intentions and weight-loss. Appetite, 74, 48-54. DOI: 10.1016/j.appet.2013.11.013

[14] Hasler, Gregor, et al., (2004). The association between short sleep duration and obesity in young adults: A 13-year prospective study. Sleep, 27(4), 661-66. DOI: 10.1093/sleep/27.4.661

[15] Gupta N. K., Mueller, W. H., Chan, W., & Meininger, J. C. (2002). Is obesity associated with poor sleep quality in adolescents? American Journal of Human Biology, 14. 762-68. DOI: 10.1002/ajhb.10093

[16] National Center for Chronic Disease Prevention and Health Promotion, Division of Population Health (2018, February 22). *Sleep and sleep disorders.* Retrieved from https://www.cdc.gov/sleep/index.html

[17] Tylkaa, T. L., Russell, H. L., & Neal, A. A. (2015). Self-compassion as a moderator of thinness-related pressures' associations with thin-ideal internalization and disordered eating. *Eating Behaviors, 17,* 23-26. DOI: 10.1016/j.eatbeh.2014.12.009

[18] Wilson, K. G. & Groom, J. (2002). *The valued living questionnaire.* Retrieved from https://www.div12.org/wp-content/uploads/2015/06/Valued-Living-Questionnaire.pdf